LUPUS
911

HOW TO BEAT
THE INCURABLE DISEASE
THAT KILLED MY BEST FRIEND!!!

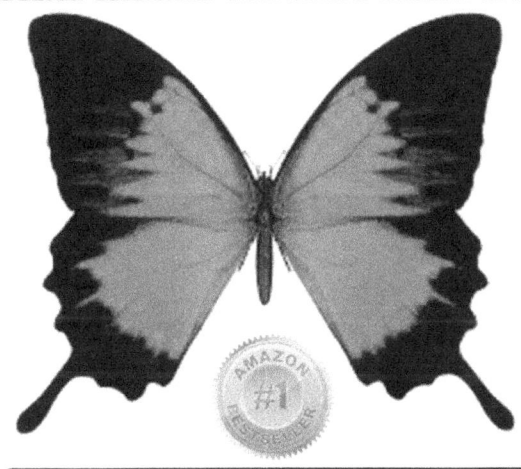

MONIC THORNTON

www.LUPUS911NATION.com

Contents

About The Author

Monic C. Thornton, is a #1 Best Selling Author and National Inspirational Leader on living with Lupus. She was born and raised in Syracuse, New York. She made Atlanta, Georgia her home after facing major complications with lupus caused by the cold and fierce winter months in New York/New Jersey that attacked her immune system, causing harm to her life.

Monic's colloquial speech reflects on the power of the mind and faith that led her to overcome critical obstacles in life with one being lupus. For many years people would always questioned the fact if lupus even existed in her body by the way she looked and her graceful spirit. Monic lives in Lawrenceville, GA with her husband Anthony and four children Toni, Kierah, Christopher, and Zachary.

About This Book

This book is written by a surviving and thriving lupus patient, who is an inspiration to lupus patients across the globe. Use this book as a guide for individuals diagnosed with lupus as well as, friends, family, and advocates who need advice on offering support. Whether you are newly diagnosed or a seasoned lupus patient, this text provides revealing material that will aid you to your wellness. With lupus being unpredictable and very complex, it can impact a person's life with no warning.

This book provides strategies that allow you to journal your own wellness. As well as, my own testimonies on how I conquer lupus each day. The advice offered allows you to set personal goals that help you to think optimistically to overcome complications with lupus.

Special Thanks To

To my heavenly Father, thank you for using me as a vessel to amplify the platform of raising lupus awareness through my personal testimony.

To my lovely daughter Kierah, because of you being born the same year I was diagnosed with Lupus, I was determined never to surrender to lupus. You gave me a purpose to live and I thank you.

To Toni, Christopher, and Zachary, you give me so much strength because of how much love and affection you show me. Your hugs and kisses help me reach for the next level with confidence knowing that you love me just as Mom at the end of each day.

To family and friends, thank you for your endless support. And, for those who are always at my bedside while in the hospital, I am forever grateful. A special thanks to my Best Friend, who is closer than a sister, Tammie, thank you for your regard, love, and support. Our friendship is a priceless gift from above.

And last, but not least, my beloved husband, Anthony, thank you for being the best husband and confidant a woman could ever ask for. I am so blessed to say that I am your wife. You have given my life more meaning. I will always love you.

#1 Best Seller Award

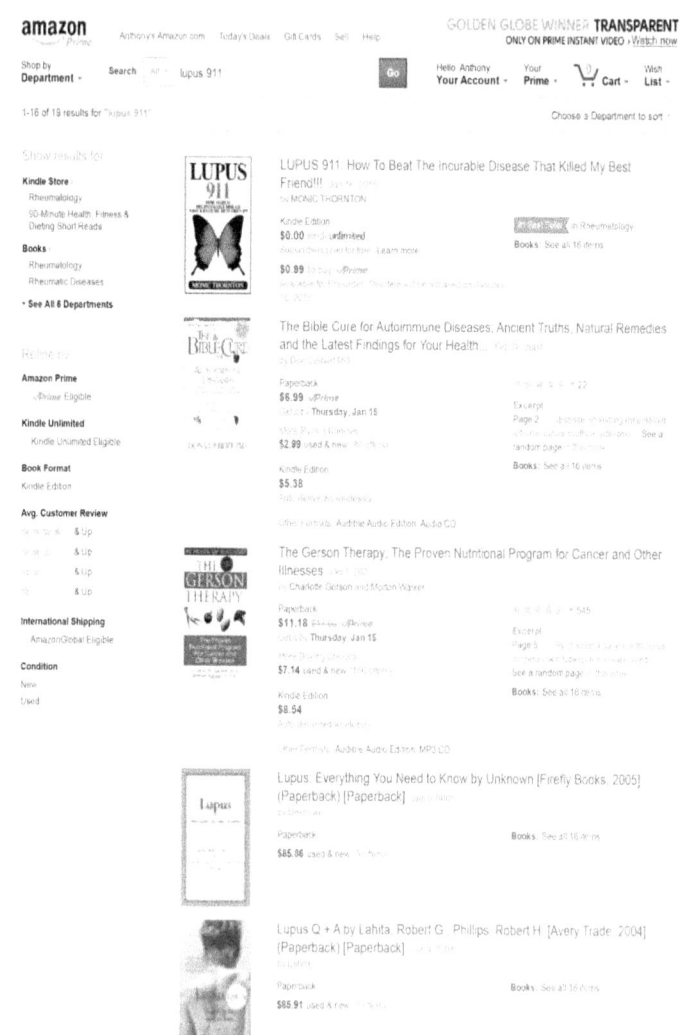

Part 1: Your Diagnosis

You Can Live!

You've been feeling really sick and fatigued lately. Your body aches, your heart is heavy, and the pain that you are experiencing both mentally and physically cannot be expressed in words. You barely have the energy to cry with your current level of discomfort. The doctors can't seem to figure out what is making you so sick and as a solution, they supply you with different types of medication hoping they'll be effective, but nothing is helping. If anything, you're feeling worse. After weeks that feel like years, you finally get your diagnosis: You Have Lupus. Does this sound like your situation or perhaps someone you know? Well, I can identify with what you're going through. At the moment, you are nervous, confused, and have many questions. You're probably wondering how and why this happen to you, especially if no one in your immediate family has the disease. Well, first I want to tell you that, *you can live with Lupus!* I know this to be true because I am writing this book, with a completely different outlook than at the time of my own diagnosis.

Like you, I had many questions and the very first being, "Will I die from lupus?" The answer is typically no, however; your quality of life will be mainly determined by your personal determination to defeat the disease. People don't die from lupus, but they do pass away from complications of the disease. You can face major obstacles caused by lupus that could affect you in a life-threatening way. The key to your survival is learning your body, remaining healthy, living a stress-free lifestyle, and having the will to fight when you want to throw in the towel and abandon hope.

I still remember the day I was diagnosed as if it happened yesterday. It was 1994 and I was pregnant with my daughter Kierah. I received a call from the nurse asking me to come into the office to discuss my blood test results. All I was thinking at that moment was what could possibly be wrong? I felt fine physically, but I entered the lobby having an odd feeling that something wasn't right. After all, good news doesn't usually require a trip to the doctor's office.

As I waited in the office, I felt like I was going to have an anxiety attack as I held on to my stomach hoping the results wouldn't cause harm to my unborn child. I walked slowly and nervously into the doctor's office, and before he could speak, I frantically asked, "Is there's something wrong with my baby?" I sat in the chair anticipating the worst as my eyes filled up with tears. The doctor replied with a calm and clear no - relief swept over me for the moment, but then why did they call me in? The doctor then began to address the findings of my bloodwork, which, felt like it took forever, to tell me that I had been diagnosed with lupus. At the time, I was so unfamiliar with the disease that I had no idea how to react. As the seriousness of lupus was explained to me, my shock turned to fear.

After shedding about an hour's worth of tears, and going through a box of tissues, I gathered my belongings and left the office. That evening was one of the hardest I can remember, I felt like my life was over. Before I went to bed that evening, I prayed to God knowing that I was going to be okay for He said "*I will put none of the diseases on you...For I am the Lord who heals you.*" Exodus 15:26. I woke up the next day feeling better than the previous day but still felt some level of distressed.

In this book, I share with you how I lost a dear friend of mine from complications to lupus, along with my own experiences - good, bad, and ugly which led me to the fabulous, yes fabulous, life I live now. This book brings you hope, guidance, and clarity regarding the misperception and unacknowledged disease called Lupus. Throughout the book, you have an opportunity to complete your own personal journal to help guide you on a path of health and wellness that will generate an explanatory dialog between you and your doctors.

According to the Lupus Foundation, lupus is a chronic, autoimmune disease that is incurable and can damage any part of the body including the brain.

The immune system protects a person against viruses, bacteria, and other potentially harmful agents known as foreign substances. In order for the immune system to function well, the system must identify foreign substances that could potentially cause harm to the body and eliminate them. Additionally, the immune system produces proteins called antibodies which fight off harmful foreign substances.

However, fighting off these foreign substances can be quite difficult for a lupus patient, because their immune system is too weak to fight these unfamiliar substances off. Unfortunately, a lupus patient's immune system becomes confused and is unable to differentiate between foreign substances and the body's healthy tissues. A simple military analogy can be used to explain the situation. It would be like the United States Army marching into the middle of New York City to wage war on American citizens; the very people they are supposed to protect. Furthermore, lupus can range in severity. So while one person's body may be dealing with the equivalent of an interstate rivalry, another may be experiencing a full-fledged civil war. Just as the severity will vary, so do the symptoms, which is why lupus can be extremely difficult to diagnose.

When I moved to Atlanta in the fall of 2000, I met a noble young lady who grew to be a very close friend. She was such a beautiful person inside and out. Our daughters went to the same elementary school and became the best of friends. She was with me during many hospital visits and witnessed many of the battles I experienced with lupus. She had never heard of this disease but learned very quickly of how dangerous it can be, as well as, how well lupus can be lived with. After years of friendship, she was suddenly faced with a life-changing event as she, like many of us, became aggressively sick without warning. Her illness started from a cold to a virus then on to unexplained sickness which led her to many misdiagnoses. Eventually, after countless visits to various doctors and specialists, my dear friend was finally diagnosed accurately with lupus. We couldn't believe it, all this time she watched me battle with complications of lupus, but never imagined that she might have to deal with them herself. Unlike me, after the diagnosis of lupus, her physical and mental health turned for the worse. Once she was diagnosed, the disease progressed to a life-threatening level almost immediately. She consistently had attacks that kept her in the hospital for months at a time. After her final hospital stay, she was released while still in an incredible amount of pain and hanging on for her dear life. At this point the lupus had taken complete control of her immune system. It was hard for her to walk and talk, that one night she tried to crawl to her daughter's room to get help. The exertion was too great, her condition had progressed too far, and she slipped into a coma shortly thereafter. Days later the doctor said there was nothing more they could do. She had brain damage and her immune system had shut down almost completely.

Lupus took my dear friend shortly after her diagnosis. She didn't have a chance to transition from a victim to a survivor. She had no defenses because she didn't have sufficient time to study lupus thoroughly to protect herself against further damage. Instead, the disease took hold and didn't let go. Not becoming familiar with your symptoms and not knowing what triggers a flare-up can be extremely dangerous, even fatal. Had my friend had the time to learn vital information, such as how the disease was affecting her body, she would have been able to put up a fight. Here's the thing about this disease, the scope of severity in lupus is very broad and it affect people differently. I've been surviving lupus for over 20 years now and my dear friend lost her life to lupus within a year and a half of her diagnosis. This is a prime example of two people with the same diagnosis, but very different outcomes.

You can't rid yourself of lupus, but you can control it to a point where you can live, even thrive. It begins with transforming your mind to the point where you dictate the disease. This task can only be accomplished with courage and willpower. If you know your life is worth fighting for then embark on this journey with me and make the decision that you will uphold your part to maintain quality medical care, an optimistic attitude, and determination not to give up on yourself so that YOU can live a fabulous life!

1. Education – learn all that you can about lupus!

2. Combat Lupus – once you conquer the education piece, gain knowledge of your body thoroughly and take note of any changes that are related to lupus.

3. Support Group – every state has various support group locations. If one is not nearby, join a prayer group. In the beginning stages of lupus, it's beneficial to visit a support group at least twice a month or as often as needed.

4. Plenty of Rest – it is imperative that you obtain a minimum of 8-12 hours of rest. When you are at the point of exhaustion, more than 12 hours of sleep is necessary.

5. Healthy Diet – there are certain foods that trigger a flare-up in lupus patients. Speak with an informed nutritionist and put together healthy meals that are appropriate for you.

Five goals I will contribute to becoming a
Thriving Survivor

1.

2.

3.

4.

5.

Who Gets Lupus?

Lupus does not discriminate! Five million people worldwide have this incurable disease and constantly search for answers that lead to a normal life. The disease is predominantly in African American women, but also common in Hispanic, Latino, Native American, Asian and Caucasian women. An estimated 5,000-10,000 of the 1.5 million Americans with lupus are diagnosed under the age of 18, and the percentage of children born with lupus from a parent with the disease is only five percent. The estimated likelihood that lupus patients will have a parent or sibling with lupus is between 10-20 percent. The percentage of men with lupus is very low at 10 percent, with 90 percent of cases diagnosed in women between the ages of 15-44.

I am the only family member of my family with lupus, and we've looked back 5 generations. There were many years of frustration and questioning why I been burdened with this disease. However, after witnessing many other's circumstances that were far worse than my own, I finally reached the point in my life that allowed me to value how blessed I am. Here I am living with lupus, my daughter is completely healthy, and observing major complications that other lupus patients have dealt with have helped me realize that things could be a lot worse. I believe the answer to why I am the only member of my family with lupus was answered when I started writing this book.

Rather than continuing with such psychological angst, I decided to accept the blessing that God is using me as a vessel for someone's survival. In my early stages of lupus, the pain I endured tested my faith, willpower, and took every ounce of energy from me. It completely changed my life and I was not prepared for the horrible damaged that was caused by lupus. After going through years of misery, I decided that lupus would no longer take control of my mind, body, and soul and that's when I started to be victorious.

If you are the only person in your family with lupus, it's beneficial not to waste your time trying to figure out why. As an alternative, direct your interests towards gaining an understanding of the disease, your body, and strengthening your mind so that you don't lose the battle you're fighting. I continue to mention strengthening your mind because it's very important to know that once you set your mind to believe that lupus will not defeat you, YOU have already won half the battle. Granted, this task is not easy to do. You are fighting the most physical pain you have ever been faced with while trying to cope with the fact that you have lupus. You may be experiencing different levels of anxiety or perhaps don't feel that you're not strong enough to survive. You can do it! In coming chapters, I will provide different strategies on how to overcome complications of lupus. Alike, give you the opportunity to track the results of your written plan to wellness.

1. Do NOT attach your identity to the disease - accept that lupus is a *part* of your life, you are so much more.

2. Denial - is normal for people after a drastic transformation or major shock. A common indicator is rejecting medicine that's prescribed by your doctor. Consequently, not taking medicine will lead to a path of destruction.

3. Resentment and fear go hand in hand. Do not fault yourself for having lupus. If you feel your condition is extreme, see a psychologist to help you manage with your disorder. The best way to reduce fear is to become educated on lupus. The more your conditioned, the more you are in control.

4. Faith – don't feel defeated by your diagnosis. It's common to assume that your condition will bring life restrictions. However, the limitations that you encounter can lead to a healthier lifestyle.

5. Success – once you are at the point of acceptance, you have really started to succeed. With success, you will develop

confidence in your ability to live a full and satisfying life, and this will help you guide others who may be struggling with acceptance.

Changes You've Made & Accepted

1.

2.

3.

4.

5.

What Are The Symptoms of Lupus?

With lupus affecting various organs, it generates a wide range of symptoms. Some symptoms are mild and temporary while other symptoms last over the course of the disease. The most common symptoms of lupus are:

Pain or swelling in the joints
Pain in the chest during deep breathing; also known as pleurisy
Extreme fatigue (exhaustion)
Headaches
Fever
Anemia
Swelling in feet, legs, hands, and eyes; also known as edema
Sun or light sensitivity
Hair loss
Abnormal blood clotting
Cold hands and feet
Mouth and/or nose ulcers

I had no painful symptoms during the early stages of lupus. I was diagnosed through the results of my bloodwork. Surprisingly, it wasn't until months after I had my daughter when I experienced the first horrific pain cause by a lupus flare up. My daughter was a newborn, and we were home alone at the time when my sleep was disturbed by excruciating pain in my body. I attempted to get out of bed to prepare my daughter's food but was unable to move because of the stiffness in my body. I finally managed to get out of bed and walked slowly to the kitchen using the wall as a clutch to keep my balance. I was unable to open my daughter's bottle because the joints in my fingers were so stiff and swollen that I could not move them at all. Actually, I wasn't able to even make a fist with my hand. I was powerless and at a standstill. After I exhausted myself with multiple tries, I eventually called my neighbor and asked her to rescue me. I was very distraught and mentally overwhelmed that day. I was supposed to take care of my baby but yet, I was in too much pain and could not physically move. Fortunately, I had a close friend that stayed in my apartment building. I managed to dial her number and desperately asked for help. My friend stayed with me for the remainder of the day and for that I will always be grateful. I couldn't imagine how I was going to care for my daughter on that particular day with the amount of pain I endured. However, it proved to be a great learning experience. I did not want to remain in such agony pain; therefore I quickly figured out that when I remained motionless, my pain was constant. Yet, when I put forth effort into moving aching body parts, the pain would come in more manageable rotations.

Now days, whenever I am faced with that type of debilitating situation, I begin my recovery process by doing light exercises such as leg lifts while lying in the bed without over-exerting myself. Each day while still in pain, I increase the quantity until I feel I have enough strength to walk. Now don't get me wrong, it's very difficult to walk while in pain, but this was a case of desperate times calling for desperate measures. You don't have to speed walk or stroll for hours. I typically start off walking for five minutes a day around the house and then increase the distance as I continue to develop strength. I never knew how well the body and mind worked unit until I began living with lupus and by committing myself to exercise. This routine, has strengthened my drive and continues to relieve me of pain in no time. In fact, I typically recover faster than my doctors anticipate, and it's all because of my determination to not let lupus control me.

Another symptom I experience from time to time is extreme fatigue. This type of exhaustion reduces physical energy and psychological ability which can become an incapacitating condition. Now, if you ask someone who see me often, they will tell you that I am extremely energetic and always have a cheerful attitude. Note, my energy derives from exercising, eating healthy, and living a vibrant life. If I lack in any of these area, my fatigue is at an ultimate high level. Furthermore, the cause of extreme fatigue in lupus patients is unclear and unpredictable but ongoing research trials are being conducted for potential treatments. Thus, important factors that contribute to this level of fatigue originate with deprived sleep, depression, anxiety, anemia, and lack of vitamin D. As a lupus patient you can control some of the contributing factors by simply making a decision to change your lifestyle and being conscious about forthcoming situations that you know causes a high level of stress. For starters, AVOID overly stressful situations if possible. If you cannot get around the circumstance as a substitute, occupy yourself in any activity that brings you peace of mind such as reading a book, watching a movie or exercising. Personally, I try to stay completely clear of negative situations and people because they are exhausting. Now, we are human and we will get upset over situations, but if you have no control over it, then LET IT GO! Remember, if you continue to stay infuriated over your situation, you are giving that incident power over you. Instead, it's better to pray about your situation and make the decision to release yourself from the absurdity.

I consider myself a seasoned veteran of lupus, I've experienced just about every known symptom and many surgeries that the illness can bring with the exception of organ replacement. The difference now, is that I'm very familiar with the disease, therefore; some of the symptoms I experienced in my early stages of lupus have reduced in severity. As you begin to experience different symptoms, it's very important for you to take detailed notes as they take place. This is a logical way for you to keep track of your condition and guard yourself from a full blown attack occurring. How many times have you suffered from a symptom that you did not write down and by the time of your doctor appointment, you couldn't seem to remember much about it? By tracking your symptoms as they ensue, you will be able to provide your doctor detailed information as to what may be causing the symptoms to occur. Remember, one of the ways a doctor diagnose you is through the information and symptoms that YOU provide.

1. Swelling Joints Pain – Wrap the affected area(s) in a warm cloth. Taking ibuprofen or a filler in your prednisone will help the swelling go down. If the swelling continues, contact your physician because it could be something more serious such as Nephrotic Syndrome, an illness where swelling is located throughout the body as well as the hands, feet, lower legs, and eyelids. A helpful indicator of this disorder is "foamy" urine.

2. Headaches –find your favorite place in the house and relax. If that doesn't work, take a warm bath because it's therapeutic and relives tension headaches.

3. Fatigue – Exercising and being active will help you increase your energy and mood.

4. Surround yourself with supportive people – Family and close friends is always helpful. Personally, I have certain family members and friends that I can always depend on.

5. Oral and Nasal Ulcers – you may experience lesions that feel like "canker

sores." These outbreaks are not threatening but can be very irritating. Using a dab of Vitamin E moisturizer on the affected area can bring some hydration and relief.

In general, keep a record of different methods that have helped you to feel better. If you are having trouble finding an appropriate healing mechanism, speak with your doctor to find other possible solutions.

Track your symptoms

1.

2.

3.

4.

5.

Different Forms of Lupus

There are four types of lupus: Systemic Lupus Erythematosus (SLE), Discoid Lupus (CLE) Drug-Induced Lupus (DIL), and Neonatal Lupus. SLE is the most common form of lupus and considered more serious and complex than the other three forms. It is not contagious and it's in no shape or form related to cancer or any other autoimmune diseases. SLE mostly harms the skin, joints, and organs such as kidneys, heart, lungs, blood vessels and brain. Systemic means the disease can affect organs and tissue in the body. SLE is considered more complex because it mimics other diseases which can lead to misdiagnosis; adding to the unpredictability and danger.

I can personally attest to this. I have two forms of lupus with SLE being one of the two. In 2004, I was in the hospital for three weeks with Pneumonia. I had a fever of 104 that would not break for seven days. They tried everything from cooling pads to large ice packets that covered my entire body. Each day became worse than the previous day. My immune system was breaking down and causing a threat to my kidneys and lungs.

One morning while I was in the hospital, I woke up in a panic because I had an IV with at least ten different medicines going into my body. Shortly thereafter, every type of specialist you can think of surrounded my bed post with a look of uncertainty on their faces. One thing about lupus, when things get bad, you are always thinking the worse because your immune system can break down rapidly. The specialists surrounding me were honest telling me that they couldn't figure out what was going on. Every medicine they treated me with was ineffective, and more importantly they could not break my fever of 104. At that moment my bloodwork was showing positive signs of Tuberculosis and my immune system was shutting down. I asked them to take me off the IV and medicines and start back from the beginning. I also requested that I be allowed to get out of bed to take short walks around the hallway to strengthen my body. I figured if this method worked at home then why not try it in the hospital. I was tired of being in the hospital and ready to go home!

During the second week of my stay, I gained enough strength to get out of bed. I asked nurses and visitors to assist me while walking the hospital corridors because I knew it would help me increase my strength. To this day, whenever I am faced with a debilitating situation, I push myself and hold myself accountable, because I strongly feel the longer you rely on someone else, the longer it takes for you to become well. Now I am not saying you don't initially need help, because you do, especially during your weakest duration which is when you first have an attack. What I am stressing is to have faith in yourself and try to do things for yourself first. Then if it doesn't work for you initially, have someone to assist you until you have enough strength to do for yourself. To review, if you should ever be faced with a comparable situation and you have the opportunity to improve functioning by yourself, you will need to push yourself through the pain (within reason) and take the necessary steps to free yourself from bondage. If you don't, you are allowing your mind to be captivated by psychological torment.

Thankfully, by the Grace of God, my vitals in the third week of my hospital stay went back to normal. My fever broke immediately, and I was re-tested. Lo and behold, all my bloodwork results that were initially positive came back negative, and I was released from the hospital. So in reality, I did not have TB and my immune system was perfectly fine with the exception of some fluids in my lungs, but because the form of lupus I have mimics many other diseases my results were misidentified at first, and I'm sure it had something to do with my over active immune system. This is why I strongly suggest that you learn your body inside and out,

because you have the potential to know your

body best.

Types of Tests for Lupus

Testing for lupus is very complex. No single test alone can determine a lupus diagnosis. For that reason, according to the Lupus Foundation of America, the most common tests used to diagnose SLE include but not limited to:

Antibody Tests - This is the initial screening test to diagnose SLE lupus. Antinuclear antibody panel is a blood test that checks for antinuclear antibodies (ANA) – having a positive sign of ANA in the blood suggests a type of autoimmune disease. 95 percent of lupus patients have a positive ANA.

Double-stranded DNA autoantibodies (dsDNA) Antibodies targeted against genetic material in the cell. Elevated levels presented in this form characterize lupus affecting the kidneys. These autoantibodies are exclusive to lupus and are very rarely related to other autoimmune diseases.

Chest X-Ray – can illustrate abnormalities – that may indicate fluid or inflammation within the lungs.

Echocardiogram- passes sound waves to generate images of the heart. This allows the doctor to examine the flow of blood by the heart beat to identify abnormalities in the heart muscle and valves.

Testing for blood disorders Complete Blood Count (CBC) –is used to measure the cell counts in the blood that include red blood cells (RBCs), white blood cells (WBCs), hemoglobin, and platelets. Having a low platelet level is a good indicator that the bone marrow may not be producing the adequate amount of platelets or that antibodies are attacking them. Most people with lupus show abnormalities in their CBCs.

Hemoglobin – is the protein inside red cells that transmits oxygen from the lungs to the tissues of the body. The amount per red blood cell (MCH) - this is comparative to the size of the cell (hemoglobin concentration) per red blood cell (MCHC). Lupus patients who suffer from Anemia, the most common blood disorder, have low hemoglobin or red blood cell count.

Urinalysis Test

Urine test are frequently requested by doctors to check for different components of urine. Urine is a waste product produced by kidneys. About 60 percent of patients with SLE will acquire clinically noticeable Lupus nephritis. This is where a lupus patient has an increased loss of protein in the urine which leads to a buildup of sodium and water in the external tissues creating edema.

Discoid Lupus is known as Cutaneous Lupus Erythematosus (CLE) and like systemic lupus erythematosus (SLE), the cause is unknown. This is the second type of lupus that I have. This form of lupus occurs in all ages and affects women more than men. CLE is a skin condition that presents itself in three main subtypes: acute, sub-acute, and chronic.

The most distinctive sign of discoid lupus is the discoid lesions. It comes in a circular and elevated lesion that's considered to be chronic. The lesions create sores by means of inflammation and scarring upon the face (bridge of the nose, around the eyes, cheeks, and ears) aka the "butterfly rash". It can also be found on the neck, scalp, and at times other parts of the body. It is critical for individuals with this form of lupus to stay clear of ultra-violet rays and the sun. During summer months it's always a good idea to wear a hat to protect your face and a wardrobe that covers most of your body. If your skin is highly sensitive, I would suggest you find clothing that has built in SPF protection. With sunscreen, it's imperative to always wear the sunblock with Helioplex and an SPF of 70 or higher. Such sunblock should be in your possession at all times. If you fail to apply the sufficient amount of sunscreen, your rashes could turn red, scaly, and possibly trigger a flare. I would also advise you to check the SPF sunscreen first to make sure the kind you have does not cause skin irritation.

During my high school years, I was that girl who never wore makeup, but things started to change as I noticed a little spot on the right side of my cheek that occurred during my pregnancy. The spot multiplied and grew into a shape of a butterfly - the naming of butterfly rash came about due to the inflammation having the resemblance of an actual butterfly which illustrates the rash crossing over the width of the face and spreading over both cheeks and bridge of the nose. Lupus is Latin for wolf; the rash extension across the face is also described as a wolf bite. Additionally, I learned later that I had Discoid Lupus and became very frantic of what this disease can potentially do to my entire body. Thus, I quickly learned that it only affect certain parts of the body. Here I was in college at Syracuse University and pregnant. I not only had to deal with the pain of lupus causing me to miss classes, the worry of my unborn child, but also, the appearance of my face that was very upsetting to me at that time. I had a huge complex mainly because people would stare at me with a curious look. This created insecurities about the way I perceived myself. At times, I hated to go outdoors because I knew the type of reaction I would get when people discovered my rash. For this reason, I thought of myself as an outsider. I knew I could not stay in this negative mind-frame too long or it would cause harm. I eventually grew mentally and spiritually stronger. I learned very quickly, educational factors that I believed would make me feel better about myself such as, my skin type and methods that I could apply that was conducive to my struggle with the appearance of my face. One of the ways I overcame the dejection was by learning how to apply makeup. Experimenting makeup techniques was a process for me in the beginning. Eventually, I became so skilled, that up to this very day, I get huge compliments from licensed makeup artists. It's amazing how knowledgeable and skilled you become when you are anxious. Now, I am more confidant that ever in my own skin and wear makeup because of my preference and not because I have a complex.

At the acute and subacute levels, non-scarring lesions are formed in sun-exposed areas such as the upper back, shoulders, outer part of the arms, neck, and the chest area. Some lupus patients are faced with severe alopecia caused by the discoid lesions on the scalp, creating massive hair loss. In spite of this, the face is often sheltered from lesions. The typical medicines used to treat this form of lupus are sunscreens, corticosteroids, and antimalarial -- treatments. Note, although this form have a non-scarring effect, it can result in dyspigmentation – a condition of pigmentation of skin or hair.

Additionally, subacute is known to have a sudden onset after affected areas are highly exposed to sunlight. The main difference between the subacute cutaneous lesions and acute cutaneous lupus is the acute form, produces the butterfly rash.

More importantly, because lupus patients face sun sensitivity, it's imperative to educate yourself on the risks caused by sun exposure and ultraviolet lights. Be aware, lupus patients are sensitive to UVA and UVB lights, and fluorescent lights which may cause skin cells in your body to die. Once the cells are dead, they produce an inflammatory reaction in your skin causing a rash to form. As a result, the UVA/UVB lights can trigger a flare-up not only causing inflammation to the affected areas, but also joint pain and fatigue, and in extreme cases such as sunburns, it can affect the muscles and internal organs. Be mindful, the ultraviolet light is at its strongest during mid-day; therefore be cognitive and stay clear of the sun during the hours of 10 a.m. and 4 p.m.

If you suffer from discoid lupus and have a complex, try not to be distraught. To bring you comfort, I am no longer faced with the burdened of a butterfly rash on my face. I was told that my pigmentation would never resurface. However, most of my skin-color returned. I do have slight discoloration, but nothing significant that would initiate embarrassment to show my uncovered face. I'll be honest, it took time to become accustomed to the butterfly rash, but I grew to be comfortable as I exposed my bare skin regularly. We as humans mull over our own appearances beyond what the general public thinks. Now don't be misguided, it took time for me to progress to this level. In the beginning, I never left my house without makeup on. Today, I am self-assured in my bare skin and have faith in my beauty, inside and out! We all have our own ways of dealing with a complex. What I want you to know is that you too are truly beautiful and we must grow to learn that beauty is only skin deep. Nobody's skin remains the same, and what I've realized, the more you're confident in yourself, the further it displays in your beauty.

Drug-Induced Lupus (DILE) is an alternative of lupus erythematosus that is uncommon and normally clears up within days to months after removal of a particular drug prescribed to an individual who has no fundamental immune system dysfunction. This type of diagnosis is triggered after a person is exposed to certain drugs such as procainamide and hydralazine, which are two of the most common drugs that cause DILE for an unremitting time. Moreover, due to DILE being very similar to SLE in clinical and laboratory features, careful consideration must be taken to distinguish between the two forms so that proper intervention is in established.

Drug-induced lupus is recognized in three groups: Drug-induced Systemic (SLE), Drug-induced Sub-acute Cutaneous LE (SLE), and Drug-induced Chronic Cutaneous LE (CLE).

Drug-induced LE (SLE) forms with a delayed start of mild symptoms. Symptoms include joint and muscle pain, fever, and pleurisy. Some individuals are affected by the butterfly rash, hair loss, mouth ulcers, and discoid rashes. This form also has an effect on organs such as kidney, nervous system, and lymph node swelling.

Drug-induced sub-acute cutaneous LE (SLCE) does not display dissimilarly in histological, immunological or laboratory elements. The skin rash that's generated is a non-scarring ringshaped rash that's normally revealed on sunexposed areas. The rash may appear on other body parts such as lower legs displayed as blisters.

Drug-induced Chronic LE (CLE) is the rarest of all three forms. It appears on the average, eight months after starting the harmful medication. This form affects men and women equally and known to affect older individuals more often. The rash has similarities to discoid lupus.

Important factors of Drug-induced LE:
It's more predominant in Caucasians.

Drugs associated with LE are given 4 categories:
1. Definite association
2. Probable association
3. Possible association
4. Recently reported

Most frequent trigger drug is high blood pressure medicine that blocks calcium. Though, high blood pressure and antifungal medicines are a very low risk.

Neonatal Lupus is the last form of lupus that affects newborns by way of maternal autoantibodies and is considered very rare. Unfortunately, newborns are also affected by the skin rash and irritations similar to sub-acute cutaneous LE (SCLE) mentioned previously. For most newborns, the rashes are non-scarring and emerge after birth. The main concern is the maternal antibodies not having the ability to fight off ailments, which are completely reliant on the mother. In neonatal lupus, the heart tissue, skin, liver, and blood elements are under attack. One of the greatest dangers newborns are faced with is congenital heart block, which can be fatal. The normal span of detecting this form of lupus is during weeks 20 through 30 of pregnancy, with week 23 through 24 being the time of highest risk. Please make note, the manifestation of heart problem in the fetus has no affiliation with the mother, it only has an impact on the child. The one upside of this form of lupus is that, neonatal lupus typically disappears during the first several months of the newborn's life.

How Is Lupus Treated?

Lupus is treated with prescription medications and various therapeutic treatments. The treatment plans will vary between each individual case and episode. Medications and their dosage are likely to change many times during a person's lifespan. In my own experience, when a major attack arises, I am prescribed with a heavy dose of corticosteroids to combat the inflammation in the affected areas as quickly as possible. As my body begins to heal, the dose is lessened respective to the inflammation. It is very important to only use corticosteroids on an as needed basis. Prolonged use of these medications in high amounts, produces dangerous side effects and can lead to additional illnesses.

When I was first diagnosed with lupus and all through my early struggles of lupus, I was prescribed 7-10 different medications. My corticosteroid (Prednisone) intake was as high as

60mg which brought significant risks and unpleasant physical changes. When taking such a high amount for an extended period of time, the physical form of the body is often altered. The face will bloat to take on a circular "moon" type characteristic. Concurrently, the body will retain water weight that will make appendages swell and can be quite uncomfortable. With that said, it is possible that you won't require such a high dose. Your doctor will only prescribe this amount of steroids if it's needed. If you do experience these types of symptoms, you should know that they are, for the most part, temporary. Your body will revert to a normal shape as you become healthy and your prednisone intake is lowered. Remember, you can decrease the chances of such situations if you make your best effort to stay on top of your wellbeing.

I have experienced many of the side effects that can come with prednisone use. I am thankful to say that today, my lupus is controlled with only

5mg twice a day. I do not suffer from aches and pain as much. I am extremely active, and I only take time off work for vacation, rather than illness. Moreover, I look forward to the day I am free of medicine, as I continue to revitalize my life.

What changes will you make to become healthy?

1.

2.

3.

4.

5.

Some of the most common medications prescribed to treat lupus are:

Prednisone - for lupus patients, this medicine is used to prevent the release of substances in the body that cause inflammation and used to suppress the immune system. Like all medication, it comes with advantages and disadvantages.

Advantages of prednisone include, regulating the function of the immune system and minimize swelling and inflammation. The disadvantage include weight gain, extreme fatigue, mood swings, and low bone density which is common for lupus patients. Take note, if you are a smoker and does not like to exercise or do not get enough vitamin D or calcium in your diet, the probability of bone loss is much greater.

Bone damage is introduced in two ways, Osteoporosis and Avascular Necrosis. Osteoporosis, causes the bone to progressively become thin. In contrast, avascular necrosis, is a weakening of the bone due to lack of blood supply. Certain healthy habits will minimize the risk and extent of bone loss such as consuming adequate levels of vitamin D and calcium.

Plaquenil (hydroxychloroquine) is another common medication that's prescribed to lupus patient and used to decrease pain, swelling, and prevent joint damage that leads to disability. Most lupus patients are able to tolerate this medicine and is normally prescribed 200mg twice a day or 400mg once a day if needed. Note the higher the dosage, the higher chances of side effects and toxicity. Plaquenil is a type of medicine that does not work right away. It is considered a slow-acting drug which may take up to two months before a person will actually observe progress and six months to experience full benefits.

When taking Plaquenil for the first time, your body may experience side effects such as nausea and diarrhea. With more severe reactions, you may experience hair thinning, skin rashes, and muscle weakness. Plaquenil is also known to effect your vision; therefore, it's imperative to share any visual abnormalities with your doctor. You should schedule an annual eye examination to avoid being diagnosed with hydroxychloroquine retinopathy, a condition that negatively impacts the cornea, ciliary body, and retina. Nonetheless, if caught early, this ailment can improve with cessation of Plaquenil.

Methotrexate is a drug that reduces pain and swelling in the joints. Individuals must take precaution due to the seriousness of side effects such as liver damage, infections, and increased cancer risks. Methotrexate can also cause birth defects which is why doctors recommend that this medication should not be prescribed while pregnant or attempting to get pregnant. Like many other medications for lupus, methotrexate takes time to build up before it becomes effective. Improvements are generally seen within the first 3-6 weeks of taking the medication. The common side effects include nausea or vomiting and abnormalities in the liver. This medicine is also known for causing hair loss and sensitivity to sunlight; therefore, folic acid supplements are prescribed with methotrexate to increase a person's Vitamin B levels while decreasing some of the side-effects caused by methotrexate.

There is a long list of medication prescribed for lupus patients depending on the severity of the disease. Remember, no two lupus patients are the same. The few medication named in this book are the most common prescribed. To remain healthy and pain-free, you must follow your doctor's order and take the suggested medication. As well as, educate yourself on the medication you are receiving. Furthermore, you will need to take detailed notes on how your body reacts to the medication. The best way I have found to do this is to keep a journal on the type of medication I take, the quantity and dosage amount, and dates I started or stopped medication. You will find this beneficial as it will help you track side effects you may encounter. Likewise, it will make it easier for your doctor to discover a solution to any problem that arises. Make sure to share your findings with your doctor. The information you provide, is a way to find out if you're able to get off certain medication. In the meantime, continue to stay committed and improve.

What side effects do you experience from your medication?

1.

2.

3.

4.

5.

You can also wrap a heating pad on the affected areas. If the pain is still present, take Ibuprofen which will help relieve some of swelling, pain, and inflammation. If these methods do not alleviate the pain, I increase my steroid on a temporary basis. Your doctor can prescribe additional dosage amount aka "fillers" when necessary.

Sharp chest pains during deep breathing also known as pleurisy is due to inflammation of the tissue layers that line the lungs and inner chest wall. You can relieve some of this pain by sitting straight up and taking long deep breaths. If the pain is persistent, contact your doctor. You may possibly be suffering from an infection. Your doctor can prescribe antibiotics to remedy the inflammation in the lungs.

Chronic Fatigue Syndrome (CFS) and Fibromyalgia (FMS) are two illnesses that are common for lupus patients and often times accompany one another. Depression is also often associated with these illnesses.

Additionally, these diseases cause severe, unrelenting exhaustion, muscle pain, mental uncertainty, and poor sleep. Pain derived from fibromyalgia is very similar to the pain caused by a lupus flare-up. To differentiate the two, a flare-up associated with lupus causes pain in the joint areas, whereas pain triggered from fibromyalgia is typically felt in the muscle.

Note, it's easy to get confused on where the pain is located because the severity of pain is very similar, however, the treatment used for each condition are different. To treat muscle spasms a muscle relaxer is typically prescribed. To treat a flare-up, anti-inflammatory medication is usually prescribed.

Prednisone helps to control a lupus flare by weakening your immune system, which is attacking the body. Your immune system is one of the most important focal point of your lupus because it is designed to fight off foreign substances in the body to keep you healthy.

Having a weak immune system allows a lupus patient to get infections more easily and more often than a healthy person. As an example, during the winter months, a healthy person can buy over the counter medication to relieve the symptoms of a cold; whereas over the counter medication will not always be effective for someone suffering from lupus.

A minor cough quickly turns into a viral infection that takes anywhere between 4-6 weeks to recover from. Earlier, I shared my story about when I was in the hospital for three weeks. This was a prime example of a minor cold that turned into a viral infection and led to

pneumonia.

1. Get at least 8 hours of sleep.

2. Drink 8-12 glasses of water a day.

3. Eat a healthy and well-balanced diet that includes fruits and vegetables.

4. Exercise at least 20 minutes a day. Increase your minutes when possible.

5. Wash your hands regularly. On method I use is washing my hands until I get to the end of singing the alphabet to ensure that I have germ-free hands.

Five goals to a healthy Immune System

1.

2.

3.

4.

5.

Lupus and Cold Weather

The most critical seasons for lupus patients to be extra cautious are fall and winter. The severe weather can lead to major consequences. Patients who suffer from SLE are greatly impacted by the weather due to the physical heat removed from the body rapidly, thereby reducing the amount of energy. This is the very reason why I moved to Atlanta.

The cold temperatures up north cost me multiple hospital visits with life-threatening potential. My condition got so bad that my doctor advised me to move to a warmer state. Now that I live in a warmer climate, I experience fewer complications and I am able to enjoy my winter holidays with my family rather than being in the hospital.

Today, I continue to be extremely careful when the weather changes from summer to fall, especially near the months of October and

November. It takes time for the body to adjust to changing temperatures, particularly when the weather changes drastically. As a precaution, in the fall I always wear weightless winter apparel to avoid an unexpected flare up from occurring, even though everyone else may continue to wear summer type clothing.

If you find your condition to be easily exacerbated by colder temperature, you may want to consider relocating to avoid life-threatening complications. The onset of cold weather causes severe joint pain which can ultimately trigger your lupus to flare up. In my most humble opinion, I believe it's best for lupus patients to live in an atmosphere that experience fewer changes in the weather climate. If you are also affected by Raynoud's Phenomenon, a condition that causes spasm in weakened blood vessels and pain in the fingers and toes, you may suffer even more. The poor circulation caused by this condition can possibly cause deterioration.

During the early stages of my lupus, I dealt with many emotions. It started with denial, confusion, anger, and I was always worried which led me to depression. Have you ever been in so much pain that the description of your agony could never convey the extent of what you were enduring, so much to lead you to silence? I have. My state of mind went through a detachment period that not only affected me financially, mentally, and spiritually, but also physically.

It was 2004, and I was experiencing a level of discomfort that was far worse than anything I ever imagined. I had pain shooting from every joint and muscle in my body and suffered from extreme stiffness. It took every ounce of energy to drive myself to the pharmacy that day. I was unable to walk around the grocery store to gather the items I needed. The pharmacist was kind enough to shop for me as I sat in the chair rocking back and forth in agonizing pain. I remember calling my best friend Tammie to express the misery I was going through. I knew she couldn't relate to my pain, but it was my way of crying out for help. I shared how I felt that I now understood why some people may resort to suicide in an attempt to rid themselves of such discomfort. That scared me. I knew I had to snap out it for the sake of my daughter and with that very thought, I focused my attention on bettering my psychological state. My depression and pain lasted three weeks. I could not get out of bed. It felt as though I was detained and could not release myself. I was financially drained from multiple doctor and hospital visits. I did not want to speak to anyone, and I even neglected my friends and family who tried to help me during my time of depression. You see, if you remain in a depression over an extended period of time, it will break down your immune system and allow other illnesses to form in your body. I could not allow this to happen to me.

Things started to change for the better after visiting a lupus support group. A young lady shared her story about how she prevailed through depression. One day while home alone, she was tired of being sick. She shut her bedroom door and yelled forcefully at the disease that was causing her misery. She demanded to be free of depression and was rescued. Her testimony was so strong that I wanted to try it, because like her, I was tired of being depressed. One day while home alone, I cried out to God, asking for his sufficient Grace. I thought about that young lady's story knowing that I no longer wanted to be in such a somber state. I shouted and demanded aggressively to the demon in my body, that I would no longer be captivated by its cruelness, and I would not accept the condition of being depressed. Praise God, I was instantly healed and relieved from bondage. From that day forward, I have never experienced depression again.

If you are dealing with depression and need help financially, mentally, and spiritually, please join a support group or talk to someone. Depression is nothing to be ashamed of and there are many people and resources to help. The financial and physical exhaustion you may be experiencing is causing your mental and spirituality to suffer deeply. Trust your inner wisdom and believe that lupus will not conquer you. The change of behavior will allow you to live an extraordinary life like the one that I live today. So start today by making the decision to challenge any negative thinking and work to maintain an optimistic attitude.

Part III: Can I Get Pregnant

Starting a Family

If you are thinking of starting a family, congratulations! I am sure you are uncertain about whether or not you can or should start a family. The answer is that you can. I birthed a beautiful, healthy girl while having lupus and she was not affected at all. I did, however, need to be extremely careful and make wise decisions that would not cause complications during my pregnancy.

It is very important to be aware that, during pregnancy antibodies in the mother's circulation are transported across the placenta into the bloodstream of the developing fetus. This process is essential because the fetus is unable to make antibodies on its own. Thus, it's completely dependent on maternal antibodies to fight infections. Unfortunately, for a pregnant lupus patient, the placenta cannot distinguish between antibodies that are helpful to the fetus and can cause potential harm to the growing fetus. For these reasons, you are considered a high-risk pregnancy if you have lupus. I don't say this to frighten you. This status is a logical alert for your perinatologist, an obstetrician experienced in high-risk pregnancies. Your pregnancy can still be healthy, as long as you do everything required of you.

During my pregnancy, I stayed clear of known risks and lupus did not pose a threat to me or my unborn child. I had a normal pregnancy without complications, and I was beyond grateful for that. Thankfully, today doctors use advanced technology that has improved pregnancy outcomes even further. If you are considering starting a family, it's imperative that you learn relevant information to starting a family while maintaining control of lupus. This process begins with proper planning and having thorough conversations with all of your doctors. A nutritionist or dietitian can help you plan proper meals. You must know there are possible complications that can occur during your pregnancy. To lower your chances, you should stay clear of drinking alcohol, smoking, recreational drugs, and limits your caffeine intake. If you are affected by hypertension, have presence of kidney disease, or a history of blood clots, these can potentially produce poor fetal outcome during your pregnancy. Speak with your doctors on ways to limit your risks.

One out of three women with lupus delivers their baby before completing their 37 weeks of pregnancy. I had my daughter during the 39th week of my pregnancy. Thankfully, she was not considered high risk, just a low birth weight at four pounds and eight ounces. As I was rushed to the hospital I experienced the same normal labor pains any other healthy pregnant woman, but then my blood pressure dangerously increased and was told there was a need for an emergency cesarean delivery. At first I was upset that I would not be able to have my baby innately, but I knew it was for the wellbeing of my daughter.

I don't remember much about the delivery because I was under general anesthesia. Apparently, I lost a lot of blood during surgery and had many blood clots that kept me in the hospital for an additional three weeks. Lupus does not prevent you from breastfeeding, but it's encouraged that you don't breastfeed if you're on particular medications that cause risk to a nursing baby. You will need to speak with your doctor to find out if breastfeeding is safe for your baby.

Part IV: Resources

A complicated disease such as lupus can be exhausting. You need a group of people in your life for encouragement and to help support you during difficult times. These groups are established to help patients manage the difficulties of lupus in an environment of understanding peers. Joining a support group, provides relief in knowing that you're not alone in your struggles with lupus. When there are others who understand your condition, a strong sense of connection and hope can build. The groups are typically coordinated by professional facilitators who may or may not have lupus. While attending meetings, take the initiative to share your own personal experiences. You never know how your experience might help someone else and vice versa.

Family members and friends are also important people to have for support. There will be moments when you're in desperate need of help. Whether it's a conversation or physical and financial assistance, it's important to build a strong support network. My support comes from many different sources. I depend on God first. I have a devoted husband who is highly educated on lupus and cooks most of our meals because he understands the exhaustion that lupus produce. His exemplary care helps relieve me of stress. Furthermore during hospital visits and surgeries, I am always surrounded by people who love me. My husband, aunt, brother, and dear close friends are always at my bedside from beginning to end, and I turn to them for strength when I am weak.

Before my husband, I had failed relationships due to the complications that were observed. The men in my past did not take time to educate themselves on the disease. Instead, they feared death was upon me that made them apprehensive. I was literally told by an exboyfriend, he had to breakup with me because he could not handle my illness and did not want to witness me dying. Initially, I was upset but as months went by, I was thankful of his honesty because it confirmed that he was not my lifepartner. You see, when people are not educated on a subject matter, they're inclined to assume the worst. Thankfully, I no longer have to face disappointments such as this because I have a wonderful husband who is willing to fight every battle with me. If you are currently go through an uphill relationship crusade, you may want to re-evaluate your situation and make a conscious decision that is best for you and your wellbeing. Sometimes, the one you think is good TO you, is not good FOR you. The life partner you need, is someone who is not in fear and willing to walk with you hand and hand to conquer lupus. When surrounded by a strong support system like this, it is easier to find the courage it takes to work through the most troubling times. I cannot stress how very important it is to have a support system in place. You might be surprised by just how significantly a support system can influence your wellbeing.

Tips for Supporters

It's difficult to describe pain. Most supporters of lupus patients are united by the fear, hope, concern, and anger due to witnessing the variations of stages a lupus person is faced with. Although people deal with illness in different ways, it's very important for supporters to educate themselves on lupus and offer the right type of encouragement. Furthermore, it's important to know the right time and place to offer support. In critical times, you may find yourself mentally and physically drained due to your efforts. Lupus patients often feel misunderstood by friends, family, and colleagues, and may be stricken by troublesome moods in times of physical or emotional angst. You should know that these emotional battles are not directed at you. Lupus patients often feel they are a burden to others. As a supporter, if you need to step aside for a while, it's okay to do so. An individual who suffers from lupus often experience an emotional battle when they're suffering. You may also witness isolation from a lupus patient. If you sense this, give the person adequate space, but do not cut yourself off entirely. When you feel that support is desperately needed, check on them more often. It will let them know that they're not alone. Furthermore, you can help during these critical times by offering assistance with other tasks such as, cleaning the patient's household or any matter that helps relieve physical stress from the patient. If you feel your support is not appreciated, you should know that it is valued. The lupus patient may have a hard time expressing it due to their current state. More importantly, the best way to help a lupus patient is by asking, "How can I help?" This can provide an effective method for helping to normalize a concern.

Given the many ways in which Lupus affects the immune system and tissues in the body, a patient will need a team of specialists to effectively monitor their wellbeing.

Rheumatologist – specializes in disease of joints and muscles.
Gastroenterologist – specializes in diseases of the gastrointestinal tract.

Neurologist – specializes in diseases of the brain and nervous system. You will visit this type of doctor if you suffer from kidney disease.

Pulmonologist – specializes in diseases of the lungs.

Cardiologist – Specializes in diseases of the heart. Lupus patients will visit this type of doctor if they are at risk of heart disease.

Dermatologist – specializes in diseases of the skin such a cutaneous lupus and will provide you with information such as the proper sunscreen to use.

Collaborating and building healthy relationships with doctors is an important part of any sound treatment plan. Your doctors will work hand in hand with you and help guide you to a path of better health. For that reason, it's imperative that you find a doctor that educates you. If you're newly diagnosed or haven't found a doctor you feel comfortable with, go to a lupus support group and ask other lupus patients about their experience with their doctors. This is a great way to find a good referral. You can also search for doctors that are board members of the lupus foundation in your area. My rheumatologist is a great fit for me. He is a lupus board member and highly knowledgeable. I have a great relationship with him, and he takes adequate time to educate me on the disease. He respects my willingness to learn, track my symptoms, and do all that is required of me to stay healthy. It makes the doctor's job very difficult and frustrating when a patient is not committed to bettering their health.

Part V: Healthy Lifestyle
Financial

Lupus can generate many medical bills that can become quite the financial burden. Multiple hospital visits, doctor appointments, prescriptions and insurance costs can add up very quickly. The burden of how medical costs can become a significant stressor, and too much stress can mean worsening conditions for a lupus patient. If you are suffering financially, implement a plan that will allow you to track your overall expected medical expenses and strategize on how your family can save money. One approach to use is avoiding high prescription cost by requesting generic prescriptions in lieu of brand prescriptions. You may also be eligible for government assistance programs. It's also imperative to select the appropriate health plan that's best suited for your condition and budget.

It was 2003, I was a single-parent trying to survive. I was having a rough winter, battling multiple viral infections causing many hospital visits. I did not have a high paying job and the little bit of money left over from my monthly bills was budgeted between gas, food, and medication. I was at the level of hitting rock bottom. I was embarrassed and did not want people to know my current state at that time. Praise God for the Angel Food Ministry. Because of this ministry, I was able to fill my refrigerator and freezer with decent food. I also got assistance from other non-profit organizations in the area. Because of the help that non-profit organizations offered, it helped me survive troubling times. If you are experiencing a tough time financially, please reach out to your friends, family, and community because they are there to help you. If you are battling with your pride, trust me, I know what you are going through. However, try not to feel ashamed. You are not the only person who seek help. Do I need to remind you of the recent recession causing major a high level of unemployment? We as a society, never know when a situation requires assistance. If it's available, tap into it.

Mental, physical, and spiritual wellbeing are the most important factors contributing to a healthy lifestyle. The quality of your life is influenced by relationships, finding peace and a sense of responsibility. Negative mood states can have a detrimental effect on the aforementioned areas, and such moods are quite common when dealing with lupus. It's important to recognize the challenges that lupus brings and to not let them make you a victim of your condition. You must increase your resiliency during the emotional and physical battles. However, this process does not happen overnight. It is a continuous path, and it's not always uphill. The most important thing is that the overall trend is positive.

Weight gain is a side effect of lupus that may interfere with the quality of physical wellbeing. Medication such as corticosteroids generates unpredictable side effects such as weight gain, high cholesterol and blood pressure, and cause blood sugar levels to rise thereby increasing the chances of a diabetes. These are all factors that can potentially make it difficult to maintain a balanced diet. Note, the steroids you intake, increases your appetite. To avoid such dilemmas, you must implement conscious strategies to maintain a healthy diet. A useful strategy to resist temptations is to purchase lower calorie snacks such as vegetables and fruit for your household. You can also have your physician refer you to a registered dietician. Another helpful strategy is exercising. This is an activity that people mostly try to avoid. However, if you implement daily physical activities in your life, it will motivate you to eat well, have energy, and inspire you to live a healthy lifestyle. This change of mind leads to conquering lupus. I personally exercise at least 3X a week. When I don't exercise regularly, I become very fatigued, I can't think accurately, and I don't feel as good. Overall, maintaining a quality life will allow you to control the complications of lupus coupled with your daily activities without fatigue or physical stress.

Complete remission can happen, but it is very rare. Remission is typically described as a period of time when the lupus patient does not experience symptoms or complications and the blood work results appear normal. Most patients who reach this status often stop taking their regular prescribed medication while in remission. However, in most cases the symptoms do reappear eventually and may differ in severity.

I have personally only experienced being in remission once while diagnosed with lupus. I had no evidence of pain, and my blood cell count was very good. It was in 1997, and I heard about the possibility to go into remission with lupus. I was feeling remarkably well, and my symptoms began to dissipate. After mentioning this to my doctor, he tapered my steroids down each visit as my lupus continued to stay controlled until I was able to temporarily stop the medication. My remission period lasted during the entire summer of 1997. It was great to not take medicine or deal with the intermittent complications of lupus. Unfortunately, by late fall I began experiencing the familiar symptoms that suggested the disease was active. Although I am no longer in remission, today I am proud to say that, I feel great compared to the pain I once endured. I am happily married, my children are healthy, I can manage the stress in my life, and the friends and family members that I am close with are highly supportive. It took a long time to get to this point, but I am here enjoying every moment of it, and I want you to do the same. I want to share my story to provide encouragement that can possibly help other's dealing with this condition to not just live, but thrive.

I cannot be sure whether or not you will have the same experiences that I encountered, but being pro-active about your health will increase your chances of remission. As you track your symptoms, you will identify what triggers a flare-up in your body, and have a better sense of what you need to do for your own wellbeing. As you experience fewer flare-ups, let your doctor known so that your medication may potentially be lowered. If you have a good doctor he/she will be honest with you and let you know if this process is something you should consider.

Final Thoughts

I hope that this book has contributed to a great awareness of lupus. Too many times have I heard people say that they have heard of lupus, but don't really know what it is. With the number of people affected by lupus worldwide, we as a society must do better to raise awareness. Thankfully there is ongoing research and better technology for early detection and effective treatment. Lupus is a disease that can be effectively managed, and with proper care, patients can lead healthy and fulfilling lives. The future of lupus research will present opportunities for new ideas and prevention that will transform the lives of lupus patients even further.

Lupus has affected every aspect of my life and being a survivor of lupus has given me a platform to increase the awareness. I want everyone to know and that they can live a fabulous life even if lupus is a part of it. To be a victor and not a victim of this unpredictable disease, you must stay away from identified triggers of flares, and become knowledgeable about your personal state along with the disease itself. Believe in yourself and push for a quality life by taking a meaningful role in your own care. If I can live well with lupus, you can too!

What To Do After Reading This Book?

Please visit my website at

www.lupus911nation.com

Medical Resources

The Lupus Foundation of America (LFA)
http://ww.lupus.org/

American College of Rheumatology
http://www.rheumatology.org/

National Institute of Arthritis and
Musculoskeletal and Skin Diseases 9NIAMS)
http://www.niams.nih.gov/

American Autoimmune-Related Diseases
Association, Inc. (AARDA) http://aarda.org/

Arthritis Foundation (AF)
http://www.arthritis.org/

American Academy of Dermatology (AAD)
http://www.aad.org/

Partnership for Prescription Assistance
https://www.pparx.org/

Reference Page

WebMD: Day2Night: Coping with Lupus; Fighting Lupus Fatigue and Boosting Energy by Ellen Greenlaw www.webmd.com/lupus.

Lupus Foundation of America. www.lupus.org/.

The Johns Hopkins Lupus Center. www.hopkinslupus.org/

NIAMS: NYI Medical Center. www.neonatallupus.com/

Prednisone:www.drugs.com/

Benlysta: http://www.benlysta.com/

Centers for Disease Control and Prevention. Chronic Disease Overview: Costs of Chronic Disease. Centers for Disease Control and Prevention Website: http://www.dcd.gov/inccdphp/overview.htm.

Callen JP, Klein J. Subacute cutaneous lupus erythematosus. Clinical, serologic, immunogenetic, and therapeutic considerations in seventy-tow patients. Arthritis Rheum 1988; 31:1007.

Iliades, Chris, MD. Medically reviewed by Pat F. Bass III, MD, MPH. Sun Exposure and Lupus: www.everydayhealth.com/

Lupus International: Nutrition and Lupus. By Tammy O, Utset, M.D., M.P.H. Associate Professor of Medicine, University of Chicago.

www.LUPUS911NATION.com

Mackillop, LH, Germain SH, Nelson-Piercy C. Systemic
lupus erythematosus. BMJ. 2007 Nov 3;335(7626):933.

www.ingramcontent.com/pod-product-compliance
Lightning Source LLC
Chambersburg PA
CBHW070827180526
45168CB00002B/758